Copyright Disclaimer

ISBN 978-1-7331413-0-7

www.a-zmindfulness.com

CONTENTS

MINDFULNESS: **A practice of being aware of the present moment with acceptance and non-judgement**. Paying attention to what is happening right now is often challenging. People spend 46.9 percent of their waking hours thinking about something other than what they're doing, and this mind-wandering typically makes them unhappy.[1] This disconnect from the present moment with focus on what happened in the past, or what might happen in the future often creates unease, anxiety, and depression. Mindfulness empowers students of all ages to become happier, more patient, attentive, and accepting by promoting social and emotional learning in the classroom and beyond.

BENEFITS: Practicing mindfulness daily and consistently paves the way for students to become mindful instead of mind-full, allowing them to gain many advantages that include:

- Improving focus, memory, processing, attention, and academic performance.
- Developing greater self-awareness through gratitude, kindness, and visualization while connecting more deeply with body, breath, thoughts, and feelings.
- Strengthening self-regulation by learning to control thoughts, actions, and emotions.
- Empowering students to be less reactive by cultivating awareness, acceptance, and choice.
- Enhancing patience and resilience as negative thoughts and feelings lose their power.
- Increasing brain mass and creating new neural pathways, contributing to mental clarity, inner calm, and an overall happier disposition.

"Being in the present moment is the happiest way to be." [2]
-Dr. Laurie Santos, Yale Instructor on Psychology and the Good Life

CHALLENGES: In our fast-paced, multi-tasking culture and technological age, people are being bombarded with information. Students encounter social, emotional and environmental challenges, leaving them feeling exhausted, distracted, anxious, isolated, jealous or depressed. As a nation we are facing a mental health crisis, with increasing stress-related illness and limited tools for coping.

- 1 in 6 U.S. children aged 2–8 years (17.4%) had a diagnosed mental, behavioral, or developmental disorder.[3]
- Mental health disorders are the leading cause of disability in adolescents.[4]
- 1 in 5 children ages 13-18 (20%) have or will have a serious mental illness. [5]
- The average attention span is 5 seconds long. Ten years ago it was 12 minutes. [6]
- Younger people have shorter attention spans than the elderly. [7]

SOLUTIONS: A mindfulness practice is like having a compass to navigate life's challenges. *Mindful Students* teaches easy to learn, fun and engaging A-Z Mindfulness strategies which promote compassion and intention towards oneself and others while improving the ability to manage emotions and strengthen academic performance. Presenting a new mindfulness technique weekly and incorporating a daily practice, keeps educators and students inspired to learn, grow, and transform throughout the school year. Practicing A-Z Mindfulness provides a welcome pause in the day as students gain valuable life skills to better manage stress, cultivate greater awareness, and become calmer, more focused, and attentive.

"From kindergarten onward, children should be taught about taking care of emotion."
-The Dalai Lama

GETTING STARTED: After completing *Mindful Students*, educators are ready to implement mindfulness in the classroom by presenting a new strategy each week and then guiding students to practice it at a consistent time each day (such as after the morning bell or recess, or around transitions). Awareness is practiced during every lesson to enhance inner calm and improve the mind-body connection. Complete each week by encouraging students to reflect and write about the experience (see Printable Journal, page 62). Over a period of time, consistent, daily practice brings positive changes to physical, mental, and emotional well-being. Remember, everyone learns at their own pace and explores in their own time and way. Resist the urge to judge or comment. If participation becomes challenging for a student, guide them to observe (without disruption). Be patient with yourself and your students. Like any athletic, creative, or academic endeavor, mindfulness is a practice where students achieve greater benefit over time. Begin each week introducing a new A-Z Mindfulness strategy to the class and practice every day by following the highlighted process and scripts on the succeeding pages.

TRANSITION IN: Ready (lights), Set (sound), Go (Mindful Body & Breath)

Dim or turn off lights, play a relaxing sound (use Insight Timer app), then students move quickly and quietly to a designated area (with chairs facing forward and feet flat on the floor, or gathering as a group to sit on the floor with legs crossed) to practice a Mindful Body & Breath.

MINDFUL BODY: Put your hands on your lap and sit up tall like a tree. Imagine roots grounding you, while your trunk is strong and uplifted. Be mindful of your senses (body still, eyes focused, ears listening and mouth closed). Focus on how your body feels and notice the space around you.

MINDFUL BREATH: Close your eyes or cover them lightly with your hands. Take a deep breath in through your nose and blow out through your mouth, making the out breath as long as possible. Imagine smelling hot chocolate as you breathe in, then blow out and imagine cooling off the hot chocolate without spilling it. Sit with a Mindful Body and practice a Mindful Breath three times.

DAILY PRACTICE: Explore an A-Z Mindfulness strategy by following the guided scripts.

*CHALLENGE: These are optional practices to explore if/when it benefits the class.

AWARENESS: (Set a timer for 1-3 minutes). Complete each lesson with Awareness. Either teacher guided (following the script, page 4), student self-practice, or a combination of both.

TRANSITION OUT: Ready (sound), Set (Mindful Body & Breath), Go (***check-in**, lights, move)

*CHECK-IN: (Optional) Ask students to share what they noticed and/or how they are feeling.

MINDFUL STUDENTS: When all 26 A-Z Mindfulness strategies have been explored, continue to practice with a mindful moment each day. Either guide students through a technique (as done before), pick a student to lead classmates in one of the A-Z Mindfulness activities, or give each student the option to practice a strategy of their choice. Students might prefer to practice a specific technique or choose a strategy based on how they're feeling at that moment. Promote self-practice and exploration when students show the maturity to make this choice.

READY, SET, GO: Transform the classroom into a calm and focused learning environment.

- A -

AWARENESS

TRANSITION IN: Ready (lights), Set (sound), Go (Mindful Body & Breath)

DAILY PRACTICE: Explore Body, Breath, and Mind Awareness.

Body Awareness

1. Close your eyes and pay attention to your body.
2. Notice if your body feels calm or restless, heavy or light, balanced or off center, hungry or full, or anything else.
3. Become aware of the feeling of clothing touching your body and air on your skin.
4. Focus on the sounds around you. Listen closely to what you hear, even if it's silence.
5. Pay attention to the sounds inside of you. Your breath and heartbeat make sounds. Listen closely to notice if you can hear them.

Breath Awareness

1. Place your hands one on top of the other on your lower belly. Become aware as it moves in and out with each breath. The breath fills the body like air fills a balloon. Feel the breath fill you as you breathe in, then empty as you breathe out.
2. Focus on the gentle movements your whole body makes with each breath in and out.
3. Pay attention to the path your breath takes. Notice if it flows easily or feels stuck.
4. Feel the cool air entering through your nose, then notice as warm air exits.

Mind Awareness

1. Become aware if you're focused on what's happening right now, or if your mind has wandered off to something that happened in the past, or might happen in the future.
2. Random thoughts often pop into the mind. When you notice this happening, bring your attention back to your breath.
3. Notice if your mind is bombarded with thoughts or if there's any space between them.
4. Pay attention to whether your mind seems calm and clear like a snow globe that's settled or cluttered and fuzzy like a snow globe that's been shaken up.
5. Focus on how you're feeling right now.

AWARENESS: (Set a timer for 1-3 minutes to practice Awareness). With eyes closed, notice your body, breath, thoughts, and feelings. If/when the mind wanders, bring it back to the moment.

TRANSITION OUT: Ready (sound), Set (Mindful Body & Breath), Go (***check-in**, lights, move)

*CHECK-IN: (Optional) Raise your hand if you feel calm. Raise your hand if you feel focused. Raise your hand if you noticed something else that you'd like to share.

REFLECTION: Complete the week with a Journal entry (print page 62).

– B –

BEE BUZZING

TRANSITION IN: Ready (lights), Set (sound), Go (Mindful Body & Breath)

DAILY PRACTICE: When we practice one-pointed concentration and focus on sounds or feelings, our minds become less active and we feel calmer and more settled. Let's train our minds to focus.

1. Close your eyes and breathe in deeply, then breathe out slowly while humming.
2. STOP humming and become very still and quiet. Pause to notice what you feel.
3. Cover your eyes with your hands and repeat steps 1 and 2.
4. Cover your ears with your hands and repeat steps 1 and 2.
5. All sound makes vibrations. We're going to practice feeling it. Place your hands lightly on your neck and repeat steps 1 and 2.

AWARENESS: (Set a timer for 1-3 minutes to practice Awareness). With eyes closed, notice your body, breath, thoughts, and feelings. If/when the mind wanders, bring it back to the moment.

TRANSITION OUT: Ready (sound), Set (Mindful Body & Breath), Go (***check-in**, lights, move)

*CHECK-IN: (Optional) Raise your hand if you feel calm. Raise your other hand if you feel energized. Raise both hands if you feel calm and energized. Raise your hand if you noticed something else that you'd like to share.

REFLECTION: Complete the week with a Journal entry (print page 62).

- C -

CLOUD MEDITATION

TRANSITION IN: Ready (lights), Set (sound), Go (Mindful Body & Breath)

DAILY PRACTICE: Paying attention to the thoughts in your mind and choosing which ones to keep and which ones to let go of is a powerful practice. It allows us to gain control over what we focus on and how we feel. When the mind wanders, it gains control over us and may lead to negative thoughts, distractions or bad feelings. When we choose to let thoughts go, we train our mind to focus and this gives us power. With practice, it becomes easier to choose our thoughts instead of allowing these thoughts to control us.

1. Close your eyes and notice what you're thinking about right now.
2. Use your imagination to visualize a white fluffy cloud above your head.
3. Practice putting whatever you're thinking about or feeling into this cloud to create some space from these thoughts and yourself.
4. Use a Mindful Breath like a gentle breeze and blow the cloud away.
5. In your mind, watch this cloud carrying these thoughts or feelings as they drift slowly away.
6. Breathe in, imagine a cloud with a thought in it, then blow out gently to let it go.
7. Repeat step 6 three times.
8. Pause to notice how you feel.

AWARENESS: (Set a timer for 1-3 minutes to practice Awareness). With eyes closed, notice your body, breath, thoughts, and feelings. If/when the mind wanders, bring it back to the moment.

TRANSITION OUT: Ready (sound), Set (Mindful Body & Breath), Go (**check-in*, lights, move)

*CHECK-IN: (Optional) Raise your hand if you feel like there is more space in your mind because you let go of a thought. Raise your hand if you feel calm. Raise your hand if Cloud Meditation was hard for you. Remember with practice you will get better. Raise your hand if you noticed something else that you'd like to share.

REFLECTION: Complete the week with a Journal entry (print page 62).

– D –

DIRECTOR

TRANSITION IN: Ready (lights), Set (sound), Go (Mindful Body & Breath)

DAILY PRACTICE: Strengthen your mind by becoming a director of the thoughts that run through it. This allows your body to feel either energized or relaxed, your breath flows more freely, and positive thoughts fill your mind making it easier to feel happy.

1. Think about an activity that you accomplished when you felt good, special, or proud. Pick something that when you did it, you felt "in the zone" and at your best. Some examples are playing a sport, drawing a picture, dancing, reading, cooking, playing with a friend or a pet, taking a nature walk, riding a bike, making music, being kind and helpful to others, using your imagination, or anything else that made you feel great.
2. Close your eyes and without moving your body, picture doing this activity in your mind. Be the director of this memory by using your senses to recreate a clear picture, making it seem real for you in this moment.
3. As this memory becomes alive, direct your awareness to the way your body feels. Pay attention to every action and detail.
4. Imagine the sounds you hear while doing this activity.
5. Notice how you feel being the director who is in control of your mind and thoughts.

AWARENESS: (Set a timer for 1-3 minutes to practice Awareness). With eyes closed, notice your body, breath, thoughts, and feelings. If/when the mind wanders, bring it back to the moment.

TRANSITION OUT: Ready (sound), Set (Mindful Body & Breath), Go (***check-in**, lights, move)

*CHECK-IN: (Optional) Raise your hand if you feel good or proud. Raise your hand if you feel focused. Raise your hand if you noticed something else that you'd like to share.

REFLECTION: Complete the week with a Journal entry (print page 62).

- E -

ENERGY BALL

TRANSITION IN: Ready (lights), Set (sound), Go (Mindful Body & Breath)

DAILY PRACTICE: Everything is made up of energy. Let's practice feeling it.

1. Energetically rub your hands together (for about five seconds) feeling the heat energy and noticing the sound this makes.
2. Clap your hands while counting together out loud to ten.
3. Repeat steps 1 and 2 twice more.
4. Separate hands with palms facing each other, elbows touching your sides, fingers relaxed with their natural curl and imagine holding a ball the size of a basketball.
5. Notice what you feel. Some people feel tingles, heat, pulsing or a push/pull, like magnets.
6. Take a Mindful Breath and when blowing out, focus on filling up the space in between your hands with air.
7. Close your eyes, focus on this space and notice what you feel.
8. Begin slowly moving your hands in and out as if you were playing with a squishy ball. Stay focused on the feeling in your hands and in between your hands.
9. Place your hands on your chest to connect with the good energy inside of yourself.
10. Focus on someone that you'd like to send good energy to and then turn your hands out to share good energy with them.
11. Place your hands gently on your head, then neck, and then belly to connect with good energy inside of yourself.

AWARENESS: (Set a timer for 1-3 minutes to practice Awareness). With eyes closed, notice your body, breath, thoughts, and feelings. If/when the mind wanders, bring it back to the moment.

TRANSITION OUT: Ready (sound), Set (Mindful Body & Breath), Go (***check-in**, lights, move)

*CHECK-IN: (Optional) Raise your hand if you felt energy in between your hands. If you didn't feel it this time, keep practicing and maybe you'll feel it another time. Raise your hand if you feel good. Raise your hand if you noticed something else that you'd like to share.

REFLECTION: Complete the week with a Journal entry (print page 62).

– F –

FIRE BREATH

TRANSITION IN: Ready (lights), Set (sound), Go (Mindful Body & Breath)

DAILY PRACTICE: Fire is fueled with air. Bodies require air to breathe and grow. We build heat, strength and focus when we practice breathing quickly and moving lots of air through our body.

1. Place your hands one on top of the other over your lower belly.
2. Breathe in slowly, then breathe out through the nose quickly forcing the breath out. Feel the belly bigger as you breathe in and smaller as you force the breath out in short bursts.
3. Repeat steps 1 and 2 while using your hands to gently press the belly inward as you breathe out quickly through your nose.
4. Practice breathing this way 10 times.
5. Inhale and hold your breath in while lightly lifting and squeezing your muscles upward, then exhale and relax.
6. Close your eyes and sit mindfully, noticing what you feel.

*CHALLENGE: Take this challenge only if you're able to do the breath in the daily practice with ease and control. Breathe in deeply, then pump the belly with 10 quick bursts while panting out through your nose. Force the breath out with rapid exhales, while gently pressing the belly in with your hands.

AWARENESS: (Set a timer for 1-3 minutes to practice Awareness). With eyes closed, notice your body, breath, thoughts, and feelings. If/when the mind wanders, bring it back to the moment.

TRANSITION OUT: Ready (sound), Set (Mindful Body & Breath), Go (***check-in**, lights, move)

*CHECK-IN: (Optional) Raise your hand if you feel energized or hot. Raise your hand if you feel focused. Raise your hand if you did the challenge and were able to pump your belly with the breath. Raise your hand if you noticed something else that you'd like to share.

REFLECTION: Complete the week with a Journal entry (print page 62).

– G –
GRATITUDE

TRANSITION IN: Ready (lights), Set (sound), Go (Mindful Body & Breath)

DAILY PRACTICE: People who practice Gratitude feel happier than those who don't. Take time to remember people for whom you are very grateful. When we practice being grateful, it makes us feel good. When we tell people that we're grateful for them, it often makes them feel good.

1. Close your eyes and think about the people for whom you are most thankful; mom or dad, brother or sister, grandparent, teacher, coach, classmate, friend or someone else.
2. Picture all the people for whom you are thankful in a "gratitude parade" in your mind. See the people that make your life better and think about why you appreciate them.
3. Focus on one person that you're most thankful for at this moment (there's no right or wrong person) and think about why you're so thankful for them. Perhaps you're thankful for what they do for you or what you do for them.
4. Imagine telling them how thankful you are for them.
5. Notice how you feel when you focus on this special person and remember how much they mean to you.

AWARENESS: (Set a timer for 1-3 minutes to practice Awareness). With eyes closed, notice your body, breath, thoughts, and feelings. If/when the mind wanders, bring it back to the moment.

TRANSITION OUT: Ready (sound), Set (Mindful Body & Breath), Go (***check-in**, lights, move)

*CHECK-IN: (Optional) Raise your hand if you feel good or happy. Raise your hand if you feel grateful or thankful. Raise your hand if you're thankful for someone in this room.

REFLECTION: Complete the week with a Journal entry (print page 62).

- H -

HAPPY HEALTHY

TRANSITION IN: Ready (lights), Set (sound), Go (Mindful Body & Breath)

DAILY PRACTICE: The mind believes what it hears. When we say something repeatedly, it reinforces the message. Tell yourself that you're happy, healthy or anything else you'd like to feel or become.

1. Connect the thumb to each finger, start with the pointer, then move to the middle, then ring, then pinky.
2. Repeat step 1 four times, while counting together: *one, two, three, four*.
3. Touch each finger, switching on every syllable as you say: *I am happy, I am healthy*.
4. Repeat step 3 twice out loud, twice in a whisper, twice silently in your mind (lips can move, but no sound comes out), then again twice as a whisper and lastly twice out loud.
5. Close your eyes and connect your thumb to the finger that feels best. Take your time to explore which connection feels best. When you find the one, be still and hold your thumb to that finger.
6. Breathe in while imagining filling yourself up with health and hold the breath, then blow the breath out while imagining surrounding yourself with happiness.
7. Notice how you feel.

AWARENESS: (Set a timer for 1-3 minutes to practice Awareness). With eyes closed, notice your body, breath, thoughts, and feelings. If/when the mind wanders, bring it back to the moment.

TRANSITION OUT: Ready (sound), Set (Mindful Body & Breath), Go (*check-in, lights, move)

*CHECK-IN: (Optional) Raise your hand if you feel happy. Raise your other hand if you feel healthy. Raise both hands if you feel happy and healthy. Raise your hand if you noticed something else that you'd like to share.

REFLECTION: Complete the week with a Journal entry (print page 62).

– | –

IMAGINE

TRANSITION IN: Ready (lights), Set (sound), Go (Mindful Body & Breath)

DAILY PRACTICE: Using your imagination, create a special place in your mind that you can visit anytime you need a break.

1. Get comfortable sitting or lying down. Close your eyes and relax your body.
2. Imagine a natural setting where you feel safe, calm and happy. Think about a place that makes you feel really good; it can be a place that you've been to or somewhere that you'd like to go.
3. In your mind, as if you were watching a movie, pay attention to what you see. Become aware of the color of the sky. Notice if there are clouds or sun, a body of water or waterfalls, mountains or valleys, flatland or hills, grassy fields or sandy beaches, flowers or trees, animals or people, or anything else that makes this your perfect place.
4. Use your senses to notice the sounds that you hear and the smells that you experience while in this beautiful place.
5. Imagine the details of what you do while visiting this sanctuary.
6. Notice how you feel when you imagine being in your special place.
7. Take a picture in your mind so that you can come back for a visit when you want to relax and feel good.

AWARENESS: (Set a timer for 1-3 minutes to practice Awareness). With eyes closed, notice your body, breath, thoughts, and feelings. If/when the mind wanders, bring it back to the moment.

TRANSITION OUT: Ready (sound), Set (Mindful Body & Breath), Go (***check-in**, lights, move)

*CHECK-IN: (Optional) Raise your hand if you feel calm. Raise your hand if you were able to imagine a happy place. Raise your hand if you'd like to use your imagination to revisit your special place.

REFLECTION: Complete the week with a Journal entry (print page 62).

- J -

JIGGLE JAM

TRANSITION IN: Ready (lights), Set (sound), Go (Mindful Body & Breath)

DAILY PRACTICE: There is a strong connection between your body and your mind. When your body feels sluggish or lazy, your mind may feel the same way. When your body feels energized and good, your mind often feels this way, too. Moving your body is a great way to feel good.

1. Stand up with space to move around safely without hurting yourself or anyone else.
2. Close your eyes or turn so that you are not facing anyone. It is easier to explore and move freely when no one is watching.
3. Take a deep breath and start to jiggle your entire body.
4. Continue jiggling everything for one minute shaking out any tightness or negativity.
5. Move freely, feeling connected to your body and letting go of stress, tension, or pain.
6. Jiggle up high and jiggle down low. Move anyway that feels good, exploring what feels just right in this moment.
7. Jiggle your knees and practice jiggling your shoulders. Jiggle your hips. Now try jiggling your hands, then your feet. Wiggle and jiggle everything like jelly.
8. STOP jiggling.
9. Take a deep breath in and hold it, then blow out and relax.
10. Sit down, close your eyes and notice what you feel.

AWARENESS: (Set a timer for 1-3 minutes to practice Awareness). With eyes closed, notice your body, breath, thoughts, and feelings. If/when the mind wanders, bring it back to the moment.

TRANSITION OUT: Ready (sound), Set (Mindful Body & Breath), Go (***check-in**, lights, move)

*CHECK-IN: (Optional) Raise your hand if you feel good or energized. Raise your hand if it's fun to jiggle like jelly. Raise your hand if you noticed something else that you'd like to share.

REFLECTION: Complete the week with a printable Journal entry (print page 62).

- K -

KINDNESS

TRANSITION IN: Ready (lights), Set (sound), Go (Mindful Body & Breath)

DAILY PRACTICE: The mind believes what it hears, whether the words are silently repeated in your mind or spoken out loud. Sending yourself positive thoughts impacts how we feel about ourselves and towards others. Practice silently repeating kind words to yourself and others, then notice how you feel.

1. Get comfortable sitting or lying down. Close your eyes and relax your body.
2. Imagine that you're looking at yourself in a mirror. Gaze into your eyes and silently in your mind say to yourself: *May I be kind, loving and at peace.*
3. Imagine seeing a person who you feel great love for and silently in your mind repeat these words to them: *May you be kind, loving and at peace.*
4. Imagine seeing a person you don't know that well and silently in your mind repeat these words to them: *May you be kind, loving and at peace.*
5. ***CHALLENGE:** Imagine a person who you don't like or who bothers you and silently in your mind repeat these words to them: *May you be kind, loving and at peace.*
6. Repeat sending kindness to yourself again. Imagine looking into your own eyes and silently in your mind say to yourself: *May I be kind, loving and at peace.*
7. Notice how you feel after sending kindness to yourself and others.

AWARENESS: (Set a timer for 1-3 minutes to practice Awareness). With eyes closed, notice your body, breath, thoughts, and feelings. If/when the mind wanders, bring it back to the moment.

TRANSITION OUT: Ready (sound), Set (Mindful Body & Breath), Go (***check-in**, lights, move)

*CHECK-IN: (Optional) Raise your hand if you feel good. Raise your hand if you feel kind, loving or at peace. Raise your hand if you noticed something else that you'd like to share.

REFLECTION: Complete the week with a Journal entry (print page 62).

– L –

LION'S BREATH

TRANSITION IN: Ready (lights), Set (sound), Go (Mindful Body & Breath)

DAILY PRACTICE: Lion's Breath is a fun way to let go of stress and stretch some of your muscles. It may look silly, but it feels good. Lion's Breath is practiced with fingers stretched and hands like lion paws ready to pounce.

1. Sit up with arms straight and fingers stretched to knees.
2. Inhale through your nose then look up towards your brow point; open your mouth wide; stretch your tongue towards your chin and exhale while making the sound *haaa*.
3. Inhale through your nose then look down towards the tip; open your mouth wide; stretch your tongue towards your chin and exhale while making the sound *haaa*.
4. Notice if it felt more comfortable for you to gaze up at your brow or down at your nose.
5. Inhale and as you exhale Lion's Breath, look at the place that feels best for you.
6. Repeat three times.

AWARENESS: (Set a timer for 1-3 minutes to practice Awareness). With eyes closed, notice your body, breath, thoughts, and feelings. If/when the mind wanders, bring it back to the moment.

TRANSITION OUT: Ready (sound), Set (Mindful Body & Breath), Go (***check-in**, lights, move)

*CHECK-IN: (Optional) Raise your hand if you feel powerful like a lion. Raise your hand if you feel energized like a cub. Raise your hand it feels good to stretch and let go of stress.

REFLECTION: Complete the week with a Journal entry (print page 62).

– M –

MINDFUL MOVEMENT

TRANSITION IN: Ready (lights), Set (sound), Go (Mindful Body & Breath)

DAILY PRACTICE: Linking movement with your breath energizes the body and calms the mind.

1. Stand up and be sturdy and still like a mountain.
2. Feel your feet connected to the ground and your body standing strong and tall.
3. Breathe deeply, feeling your body gently sway with each breath in and out.
4. Extend your arms overhead and reach upward. Breathe in and notice how your body moves.
5. Breathe out, while slowly moving your hands together and lowering them down so that your thumbs touch the center of your chest while you bend your knees and pretend to sit in a chair.
6. Repeat steps 4 and 5 three times while linking your breath with this fluid motion.
7. Practice moving in other ways to explore the body-breath connection. Extend your arms upward as you breathe in, then fold forward as you breathe out; extend your arms up as you breathe in, then stretch over to the side as you breathe out; repeat extending up as you breath in, then stretching over to the other side as you breath out.
8. Sit down, close your eyes and become still.
9. Notice how you feel.

AWARENESS: (Set a timer for 1-3 minutes to practice Awareness). With eyes closed, notice your body, breath, thoughts, and feelings. If/when the mind wanders, bring it back to the moment.

TRANSITION OUT: Ready (sound), Set (Mindful Body & Breath), Go (***check-in**, lights, move)

*CHECK-IN: (Optional) Raise your hand if you feel calm. Raise your hand if you feel focused or energized. Raise your hand if you noticed something else that you'd like to share.

REFLECTION: Complete the week with a Journal entry (print page 62).

- N -

NOTE TO SELF

DAY 1: Read *Note to Self* (below) to class. Then students fill in *Note to Self* (print page 60).
DAILY PRACTICE: (Day 2-5) Students silently read their *Note to Self*, followed with:
TRANSITION, AWARENESS, TRANSITION, CHECK-IN, and **REFLECTION** (print page 62).

Dear Self,

I am special and perfect just the way I am. Sometimes I make mistakes, but I learn from them and am working to be the best that I can be. Each day is a gift filled with challenges and opportunities to learn and grow. When things seem hard, I remember to be my own best friend by being patient, kind, and forgiving with myself and others. I make time to do things that make me happy and feel good. I love myself and deserve to be happy!

This is why I'm special:
I am special because I am a good teacher and a great listener.

An important person to me is <u>my mom</u>. I feel this way because:
She is my best friend and is always there for me.

When this person makes a mistake, I can say this to help them feel better:
It will be okay. Everyone makes mistakes. We can learn from our mistakes. I still love you.

When I make a mistake, I will practice saying these words to myself to feel better:
It will be okay. Everyone makes mistakes. We can learn from our mistakes. I still love you.

When I do something well, I will practice saying this to myself:
I am so proud of you. You worked hard and did a great job!

I feel best when I do (list activities):
I feel best when biking, playing music, dancing, drumming, hiking, in nature, hugging, and teaching.

I am grateful for:
I am so thankful for my family, friends, and students.

With kindness, love, appreciation, and gratitude,
Lani

– O –

OCEAN BREATH

TRANSITION IN: Ready (lights), Set (sound), Go (Mindful Body & Breath)

DAILY PRACTICE: The sound and motion of the ocean can be very relaxing. Practicing Ocean Breath allows us to slow down and connect with the sound and feeling of our breath.

1. Inhale through your nose then exhale slowly through an open mouth making the ocean sound *haaa*.
2. Close your eyes and practice ocean breath again. This time imagine that you're listening to the sound of the waves. Repeat three times.
3. Practice Ocean Breath again while noticing your body moving like a wave, rising and falling with each breath in and out.
4. Move your hands upward like a wave crest as you breathe in, then let your hands flow downward like a wave rolling into the seashore as you breathe out making the ocean sound *haaa*. Repeat three times.
5. Breathe naturally, noticing how you feel when the ocean gets calm and quiet.
6. With your eyes closed, notice the soothing motion of the ocean as your body gently rises and falls with each natural breath.

*CHALLENGE: Practice Ocean Breath leaving your mouth closed. Inhale through your nose, then with lips sealed, exhale slowly while whispering the sound of *haaa*. Repeat three times.

AWARENESS: (Set a timer for 1-3 minutes to practice Awareness). With eyes closed, notice your body, breath, thoughts, and feelings. If/when the mind wanders, bring it back to the moment.

TRANSITION OUT: Ready (sound), Set (Mindful Body & Breath), Go (***check-in**, lights, move)

*CHECK-IN: (Optional) Raise your hand if you feel calm. Raise your hand if you feel focused. Raise your hand if this breath reminds you of the sound or motion of the ocean. Raise your hand if you noticed something else that you'd like to share.

REFLECTION: Complete the week with a Journal entry (print page 62).

- P -

PATTING

TRANSITION IN: Ready (lights), Set (sound), Go (Mindful Body & Breath)

DAILY PRACTICE: Patting is like a gentle self-massage that energizes the body. Be kind to yourself by patting lightly so that it feels good. Patting is a way to take care of your body and let go of stress.

1. Imagine that you're patiently waiting for it to start raining.
2. With your hands open, gently begin patting your thighs (about 5 seconds on each body part), then move to your belly and then up to your chest, as you listen to the sound and feel the pitter patter of the rain. STOP.
3. Close eyes and rest your hands in lap.
4. Take a deep breath and notice what you're feeling.
5. Use your finger tips to begin lightly patting your head, neck, eyebrows, temples, cheeks, jaw, upper lip, and chin crease. STOP.
6. Close your eyes and rest your hands in lap.
7. Take a deep breath and notice the calm, peaceful feeling after the rainstorm.
8. Notice how you feel.

AWARENESS: (Set a timer for 1-3 minutes to practice Awareness). With eyes closed, notice your body, breath, thoughts, and feelings. If/when the mind wanders, bring it back to the moment.

TRANSITION OUT: Ready (sound), Set (Mindful Body & Breath), Go (***check-in**, lights, move)

*CHECK-IN: (Optional) Raise your hand if you feel calm. Raise your hand if you feel energized. Raise your hand if patting your body makes you feel good.

REFLECTION: Complete the week with a Journal entry (print page 62).

– Q –

QUEEN SNAKE

TRANSITION IN: Ready (lights), Set (sound), Go (Mindful Body & Breath)

DAILY PRACTICE: Queen Snake cools your body down while calming your mind. Queen Snake hisses and then becomes quiet and still.

1. Form your lips into an "O". Curl your tongue lengthwise and slide it out of your mouth.
2. Inhale through your tongue, into your mouth as if your tongue is a straw sucking in air.
3. Slide your tongue back into your mouth, then hiss by pushing air out through your teeth as you exhale completely.
4. Repeat steps 1-3 while focusing on the cool sensation as you sip air in through your curled tongue. Listen to the hissing sound as air pushes out through your teeth.
5. Repeat steps 1-3 while feeling your belly fill with air that is sipped in through your curled tongue. Then hissing out through your teeth, notice as your belly empties.
6. Close your eyes and notice what you feel.

AWARENESS: (Set a timer for 1-3 minutes to practice Awareness). With eyes closed, notice your body, breath, thoughts, and feelings. If/when the mind wanders, bring it back to the moment.

TRANSITION OUT: Ready (sound), Set (Mindful Body & Breath), Go (***check-in**, lights, move)

*CHECK-IN: (Optional) Raise your hand if you feel quiet. Raise your hand if your body temperature feels cool or your mind feels calm. Raise your hand if you noticed something else that you'd like to share.

REFLECTION: Complete the week with a Journal entry (print page 62).

- R -

RELAXATION

TRANSITION IN: Ready (lights), Set (sound), Go (Mindful Body & Breath)

DAILY PRACTICE: It feels good to relax while following a full body relaxation. During this activity, you'll hear the same phrase repeated several times, instructing you to relax different parts of your body. We'll start with your toes and slowly work up to your head.

1. Get comfortable sitting or lying down. Close your eyes and relax your body.
2. Practice keeping your body still and eyes closed as you listen:

   Breathe in deeply while bringing awareness to your <u>toes</u>, breathe out completely and relax them.

3. (Substitute the listed body parts in the phrase above): <u>feet</u>, <u>ankles</u>, <u>lower legs</u>, <u>knees</u>, <u>upper legs</u>, <u>hips</u>, <u>lower belly and back</u>, <u>ribs and side body</u>, <u>chest and upper back</u>, <u>fingers</u>, <u>hands</u>, <u>lower arms</u>, <u>elbows</u>, <u>upper arms</u>, <u>shoulders</u>, <u>neck</u>, <u>face</u>, <u>eyes</u>, <u>ears</u>, and <u>skull and head</u>.
4. Take a final deep breath. Breathe in slowly while filling up with air and expanding the whole body; pause while holding the breath in then blow the breath out and relax. Let go completely.
5. Let your body be heavy and still as you relax.

AWARENESS: (Set a timer for 1-3 minutes to practice Awareness). With eyes closed, notice your body, breath, thoughts, and feelings. If/when the mind wanders, bring it back to the moment.

TRANSITION OUT: Ready (sound), Set (Mindful Body & Breath), Go (***check-in**, lights, move)

*CHECK-IN: (Optional) Raise your hand if your body feels relaxed. Raise your hand if your mind feels calm. Raise your hand if you feel tired.

REFLECTION: Complete the week with a Journal entry (print page 62).

- S -

SQUEEZE/RELEASE

TRANSITION IN: Ready (lights), Set (sound), Go (Mindful Body & Breath)

DAILY PRACTICE: When the body is feeling stressed or holding tension, the mind feels this way too. As the body relaxes, the mind is soothed and becomes calmer.

1. Get comfortable sitting or lying down. Close your eyes and relax your body.
2. Breathe in deeply and hold your breath while squeezing every muscle in your body (hands into fists, toes, legs, arms, seat, belly, back, face-eyes, lips, jaw).
3. Breathe out while making a whooshing sound through your mouth and release everything.
4. Repeat steps 2 and 3 three times.
5. Sit still and notice as your muscles relax and tension melts away.

AWARENESS: (Set a timer for 1-3 minutes to practice Awareness). With eyes closed, notice your body, breath, thoughts, and feelings. If/when the mind wanders, bring it back to the moment.

TRANSITION OUT: Ready (sound), Set (Mindful Body & Breath), Go (***check-in**, lights, move)

*CHECK-IN: (Optional) Raise your hand if your body feels relaxed. Raise your hand if your mind is calm. Raise your hand if you noticed something else that you'd like to share.

REFLECTION: Complete the week with a Journal entry (print page 62).

- T -

TAKE 5

TRANSITION IN: Ready (lights), Set (sound), Go (Mindful Body & Breath)

DAILY PRACTICE: Take 5 breath is a way to take a pause when you feel you need a break.

1. Hold your hand up like a stop sign.
2. Count using your fingers to keep track. Start by moving your thumb, then pointer, middle finger, ring finger, and pinky as you quietly say in your mind: *one, two, three, four, five.*
3. Follow step 2, while breathing in for a count of five. Next, hold your breath for a count of five. Finally, slowly blow your breath out through your mouth for a count of five.
4. Repeat three times.
5. Notice how you feel.

*CHALLENGE: Breathe in for a count of five, then hold the breath for a count of five, then slowly blow the breath out through your mouth for a count of five. Now challenge yourself by practicing holding your breath out while pausing for a count of five before breathing in again. Repeat three times.

AWARENESS: (Set a timer for 1-3 minutes to practice Awareness). With eyes closed, notice your body, breath, thoughts, and feelings. If/when the mind wanders, bring it back to the moment.

TRANSITION OUT: Ready (sound), Set (Mindful Body & Breath), Go (***check-in**, lights, move)

*CHECK-IN: (Optional) Raise your hand if you feel calm. Raise your hand if breathing this way gave your mind and body a break. Raise your hand if it's challenging to pause when holding the breath out. Raise your hand if you noticed something else that you'd like to share.

REFLECTION: Complete the week with a Journal entry (print page 62).

- U -

UNICORN WITH UJJAYI BREATH

TRANSITION IN: Ready (lights), Set (sound), Go (Mindful Body & Breath)

DAILY PRACTICE: Becoming aware of the breath while slowing it down and linking it with motion, allows your body to relax and your mind to focus.

1. Practice Ocean Breath with a closed mouth, making the sound of *haaa* on the exhale.
2. Bring your hands together palm to palm, then place your thumbs at the point in between your eye brows to make a unicorn horn.
3. With your thumbs on your forehead breathe in and then Ocean Breath out as you slide your thumbs down to the center of your chest. Repeat three times.
4. Repeat step 3 again; this time focus on the sound of your breath guiding this motion.
5. Close your eyes and notice how you feel.

*CHALLENGE: Ujjayi Breath sounds like the ocean when breathing both in and out. Practice this with your mouth closed while making the sound *haaa* as you breathe in and out. Practice Unicorn with Ujjayi Breath, sliding your thumbs down to the center of your chest with each exhale. Repeat three times.

AWARENESS: (Set a timer for 1-3 minutes to practice Awareness). With eyes closed, notice your body, breath, thoughts, and feelings. If/when the mind wanders, bring it back to the moment.

TRANSITION OUT: Ready (sound), Set (Mindful Body & Breath), Go (***check-in**, lights, move)

*CHECK-IN: (Optional) Raise your hand if you feel calm. Raise your hand if you feel focused. Raise your hand if this was challenging for you. It may take time and practice to do Ujjayi Breath with ease. Raise your hand if you noticed something else that you'd like to share.

REFLECTION: Complete the week with a Journal entry (print page 62).

– V –

VISION

"Whatever the mind can conceive and believe, the mind can achieve."
-Napoleon Hill, author Think and Grow Rich

TRANSITION IN: Ready (lights), Set (sound), Go (Mindful Body & Breath)

DAILY PRACTICE: A clear vision directs us where we're going and who we'd like to become. Believe you can achieve, then work hard to make your vision real. With a clear, creative and flexible vision, combined with lots of hard work, you can and will accomplish anything.

1. If you don't know where you're going and have a plan to get there, you surely won't arrive. Create a vision in your mind of your future self. Picture what you'd like to do and who you'd like to become.
2. Close your eyes and in your mind see the way you'd like your life to be. Focus on what's most important to you. Visualize being happy with family, friends and at school. Imagine that you can achieve anything and that no one or nothing can stop you. Picture yourself doing fun, challenging or creative activities with ease and grace.
3. This is your vision. See yourself doing these things well while surrounded by the people who are most important to you.
4. Let go of any thoughts that might hold you back or prevent you from achieving your vision. You are the superstar of your vision. See it clearly as if you were watching a movie in your mind. Visualize what you'd like to do or be and see yourself becoming this superstar.
5. Notice how you feel.

AWARENESS: (Set a timer for 1-3 minutes to practice Awareness). With eyes closed, notice your body, breath, thoughts, and feelings. If/when the mind wanders, bring it back to the moment.

TRANSITION OUT: Ready (sound), Set (Mindful Body & Breath), Go (***check-in**, lights, move)

*CHECK-IN: (Optional) Raise your hand if you feel clear about where you're going and who you'd like to be. Raise your hand if you noticed something else that you'd like to share.

REFLECTION: Complete the week with a Journal entry (print page 62).

– W –

WATER

TRANSITION IN: Ready (lights), Set (sound), Go (Mindful Body & Breath)

DAILY PRACTICE: A calm mind is like smooth, peaceful, clear water. Thoughts are like rocks that create ripples, take up space and disturb the peace. Many thoughts clutter the mind and leave us feeling restless or weighed down.

1. Close your eyes and imagine seeing calm, still water.
2. Visualize a rock being dropped into the water. Imagine this rock creating ripples that go on and on, disturbing the stillness.
3. Imagine another rock being dropped into the water, then in your mind watch it sinking slowly down to the bottom, settling next to other rocks that are down there. Rocks take up space and clutter the clear water. Rocks in the water can get in the way or be harmful.
4. Take a Mindful Breath and as you blow out, imagine a strong current washing away all the rocks and creating more space.
5. Visualize clear, calm, soothing, still water again.
6. Practice a Mindful Breath to wash away any thoughts in your mind that don't serve you; imagine the clutter in your mind floating away.
7. Notice how you feel with your mind clear and calm, like smooth water.

AWARENESS: (Set a timer for 1-3 minutes to practice Awareness). With eyes closed, notice your body, breath, thoughts, and feelings. If/when the mind wanders, bring it back to the moment.

TRANSITION OUT: Ready (sound), Set (Mindful Body & Breath), Go (***check-in**, lights, move)

*CHECK-IN: (Optional) Raise your hand if you feel calm. Raise your hand if you noticed any thoughts creating ripples in your mind. Raise your hand if you noticed something else that you'd like to share.

REFLECTION: Complete the week with a Journal entry (print page 62).

- X -

X-TRAORDINARY YOU

TRANSITION IN: Ready (lights), Set (sound), Go (Mindful Body & Breath)

DAILY PRACTICE: No one else is just like you. Each person is different and unique. You are special just the way you are. Remember who you are and where you came from. When you feel down or lonely, remember that you are extraordinary and loved. Strive to be the best version of yourself. Become a person that you feel proud of and who you like. You deserve to do things that make you happy and feel good. You are loved, special, and X-traordinary!

1. Cross your arms like an X and give yourself a big hug.
2. Close your eyes and send yourself kindness, love, and peace.
3. Focus on what you like best about yourself.
4. Think about what you're good at; something that when you do it you feel your best.
5. Remember a time when you accomplished something and felt proud.
6. Focus on what you like about how you look, act, and think.
7. Think about what makes you a good friend to others.
8. Think about what makes you a great friend to yourself.
9. Visualize everything and anything that you like best about YOU.

AWARENESS: (Set a timer for 1-3 minutes to practice Awareness). With eyes closed, notice your body, breath, thoughts, and feelings. If/when the mind wanders, bring it back to the moment.

TRANSITION OUT: Ready (sound), Set (Mindful Body & Breath), Go (***check-in**, lights, move)

*CHECK-IN: (Optional) Raise your hand if you feel special. Raise your hand if you're a good friend. Raise your hand if you'd like to be your own best friend. Raise your hand if you noticed something else that you'd like to share.

REFLECTION: Complete the week with a Journal entry (print page 62).

- Y -

YELLOW MELLOW

TRANSITION IN: Ready (lights), Set (sound), Go (Mindful Body & Breath)

DAILY PRACTICE: The words of this song express Yellow Mellow:

> *"May the long-time sun shine upon you, all love surround you*
> *and the pure light within you, guide your way on."* [8]
> *-Mike Heron from the Incredible String Band*

1. Imagine the bright sun is shining warm golden rays down on you.
2. Picture this radiant, glowing light shining down through the top of your head and moving slowly to your forehead, throat, chest, belly, hips, and then flowing like liquid gold down through your legs and feet.
3. Breathe in and imagine golden, radiant energy rising up from your feet to your head; surrounding your body like a cocoon, then connecting back up to the magnificent sun.
4. Breathe out and imagine Yellow Mellow rays flowing down from your head to your toes.
5. Repeat step 3 and 4 three times.

AWARENESS: (Set a timer for 1-3 minutes to practice Awareness). With eyes closed, notice your body, breath, thoughts, and feelings. If/when the mind wanders, bring it back to the moment.

TRANSITION OUT: Ready (sound), Set (Mindful Body & Breath), Go (***check-in**, lights, move)

*CHECK-IN: (Optional) Raise your hand if you feel good. Raise your hand if you feel like Yellow Mellow glowing sunshine. Raise your hand if you noticed something else that you'd like to share.

REFLECTION: Complete the week with a Journal entry (print page 62).

- Z -

ZEN "I AM"

TRANSITION IN: Ready (lights), Set (sound), Go (Mindful Body & Breath)

DAILY PRACTICE: The mind believes what it hears, whether its words spoken out loud or thoughts silently repeated to yourself. With each letter of the alphabet, there are positive Zen "I Am" words to express who I am right now, or who I choose to become.

1. Listen as I read these words: *"I am"* ... *aware, brave, creative, determined, energetic, funny, grateful, happy, healthy, humble, intelligent, important, joyful, kind, loving, mindful, nice, observant, patient, peaceful, qualified, radiant, special, thankful, unique, vivacious, wise, x-traordinary, youthful and Zen.*
2. Close your eyes and notice how you feel after hearing these words.
3. Focus on words that describe who you are now or who you'd like to become.
   Remember that having a clear plan for what you'd like to do and who you'd like to become is the best way to get there. In your mind, silently say to yourself, Zen "I am" and fill it in with all that you are or all that you'd like to be.

*CHALLENGE: Practice finding words that begin with each letter of the alphabet that describe who you are now or who you'd like to become.

AWARENESS: (Set a timer for 1-3 minutes to practice Awareness). With eyes closed, notice your body, breath, thoughts, and feelings. If/when the mind wanders, bring it back to the moment.

TRANSITION OUT: Ready (sound), Set (Mindful Body & Breath), Go (***check-in**, lights, move)

*CHECK-IN: (Optional) Raise your hand if you feel good. Raise your hand if you feel special. Everyone should have a hand up because you're all special. Raise both hands high because you're very special. Leave hands up if you'd like to share words that describe you or who you'd like to become.

REFLECTION: Complete the week with a Journal entry (print page 62).

NOTE TO SELF (PRINTABLE)

Dear Self,

I am special and perfect just the way I am. Sometimes I make mistakes, but I learn from them and am working to be the best that I can be. Each day is a gift filled with challenges and opportunities to learn and grow. When things seem hard, I remember to be my own best friend by being patient, kind, and forgiving with myself and others. I make time to do things that make me happy and feel good. I love myself and deserve to be happy!

This is why I'm special:

An important person to me is _____. I feel this way because:

When this person makes a mistake, I can say this to help them feel better:

When I make a mistake, I will practice saying these words to myself to feel better:

When I do something well, I will practice saying this to myself:

I feel best when I do (list activities):

I am grateful for:

With kindness, love, appreciation and gratitude,

JOURNAL (PRINTABLE)

When I practice this A-Z Mindfulness activity_____, I notice...

My body feels_____

This tells me_____

My breath feels_____

This tells me_____

The thoughts in my head_____

This tells me_____

I feel _____

This tells me_____

A good time to practice this activity is _____

*CHALLENGE (Optional): Circle each day that you practiced this activity on your own.

M   T   W   Th   F   S   Su

Draw picture or journal (on back)

TESTIMONIALS

"I love 'Ocean Breath.' It makes me feel calm. I will do deep breathing at my house."
-Henry, 1st grader

"We learned how to think about our positive feelings. We also learned how to take away bad feelings and thoughts. We enjoyed 'Take 5,' it helped calm our bodies."
-2nd grade class, Cherokee

"'Jiggle Jam' makes my body active then calm. I feel happy and am having fun because I'm 'Fire-working' stress ott. It's active and lets ott unhappiness. I can practice when I have thoughts to let out."
-3rd grader, Northbrook

"When I practice 'Awareness,' I am aware of my surroundings. My body is calm and collected and my breath is slow and relaxed. I feel great and ready for anything because I am calm and aware. I can practice after school and before homework."
-Maya, 4th grader

"I've noticed that students show better decision making, not so quick to blame peers."
-Schlemm, 4th grade teacher

"I enjoyed learning about mindfulness and trying all the techniques. I liked acting out each technique and practicing with peers. I've practiced going to my ideal space, creating a stress cloud and blowing it away."
-11th grade, Schuler Scholar

"Students were engrossed in instruction and continued to talk about practices throughout the day. I love continuing to focus on 'Awareness' this week and journaling Friday."
-2nd grade teacher, Hickory Point

"Breathing techniques help students relax. The kids like them and thought they worked."
-3rd grade teacher, Lake Forest

"Students learned valuable tools to help them deal with real life situations and so many ways to stay focused and calm."
-Bricker, 1st grade teacher

"When I practice 'X-traordinary' my mind is focused on things that I've accomplished, not things that I need to do. I think positively about myself. This makes me feel awesome, complete, happy, unique, and really good about myself."
-6th grader

"Mindfulness is a skill that the kids will use for the rest of their lives. The kids love it."
-John, P.E. Teacher

"Our favorite strategies to help us stay mindful were 'Energy Ball' and 'Imagine.' We will use these all year!"
-1st grade teacher, Room 11

"After 'Zen I am', I realized there's a lot I like about myself and times I've used 'Imagination' to relax myself in my very hectic life, it really helps!"
-Jodi Max, Teacher Children's Center Lakeside

"I realized that I can be in a relaxed state, what a nice feeling it is! This is something I can practice on my own for a short period of time each day. My mental health deserves it, I deserve it!"
-Amy Young, Teacher Children's Center Lakeside

NOTES

1. Bradt, Steve. "Wandering Mind Not a Happy Mind." Harvard Gazette. May 02, 2019. Accessed June 12, 2019. https://news.harvard.edu/gazette/story/2010/11/wandering-mind-not-a-happy-mind/.

2. "Mental Health Conversation at KO Addresses Addiction, Anxiety, and Mental Illness - We-Ha | West Hartford News." We. May 21, 2019. Accessed June 12, 2019. https://we-ha.com/mental-health-conversation-at-ko-addresses-addiction-anxiety-and-mental-illness/.

3. "Health Care, Family, and Community Factors Associated with Mental, Behavioral, and Developmental Disorders and Poverty Among Children Aged 2–8 Years - United States, 2016 | MMWR." Centers for Disease Control and Prevention. Accessed June 12, 2019. https://www.cdc.gov/mmwr/volumes/67/wr/mm6750a1.htm.

4. "Mental Health Research." Behavioral and Mental Health Research - On Our Sleeves. Accessed June 12, 2019. https://www.nationwidechildrens.org/giving/on-our-sleeves/research.

5. "NAMI." NAMI. Accessed June 12, 2019. https://www.nami.org/learn-more/mental-health-by-the-numbers.

6. Gaille, Brandon. "17 Average Attention Span Statistics and Trends." *BrandonGaille.com*, 23 May 2017. https://brandongaille.com/average-attention-span-statistics-and-trends/.

7. Gaille, Brandon. "17 Average Attention Span Statistics and Trends." *BrandonGaille.com*, 23 May 2017. https://brandongaille.com/average-attention-span-statistics-and-trends/.

8. "May the Long Time Sun Shine Upon You...Where It All Began." 3HO. March 23, 2019. Accessed June 13, 2019. https://www.3ho.org/3ho-lifestyle/healthy-happy-holy-lifestyle/about-3ho/may-long-time-sun-shine-upon-youwhere-it-all.

CPSIA information can be obtained
at www.ICGtesting.com
Printed in the USA
FFHW010252300819
54478924-60175FF